Health Benefits of Neem from the Abaco Neem Farm

Pamela Paterson

☙❧

Copyright this edition © 2012 by Pamela Paterson (www.writertypes.com)

All rights reserved. No part of this publication may be reproduced, stored in a retrieval system, or transmitted, in any form, or by any means, electronic, mechanical, photocopying, recording, or otherwise, with the prior permission in writing of the copyright holder.

ISBN: 978-1479174010

Design by Rhys Griffiths

Cover by Designisgrowth, www.designisgrowth.com

Edited by Robert Long

Contents

Preface **5**
   Note to Reader 5
Chapter 1: Introduction **7**
Chapter 2: Abaco Neem Story **9**
   Starting the Farm 9
   Abaco Neem Farm Today 10
Chapter 3: About the Neem Tree **11**
   Habitat—Dry, Hot, and Sunny 11
   Chemistry of Neem 13
Chapter 4: Safety of Neem **15**
Chapter 5: Remedies by Health Topic **17**
   List of Neem Remedies by Health Topic 17
Chapter 6: Select Health Issues **27**
   Chemical Complexity of Neem 27
   Antioxidant 27
   Cancer 28
   Dental and Oral Care 28
   Diabetes 29
   HIV/AIDS 29
   Pregnancy and Contraception 29
   Skin Disorders 29

Contents

    Ulcers 30

Chapter 7: Pet Health Benefits 31
    Remedies by Pet Health Topic 32

Chapter 8: Enviro- and Agri-Benefits 33
    Erosion Control 33
    Soil Enhancer 33
    Parasite Control 33
    Pesticide—Gentle and Safe 34
    Citrus Tree Pest Reduction 34
    A Future with Less Harmful Pesticides? 35
    Using Neem as a Pesticide in Your Home 35

Chapter 9: Learning More 37

Appendix A Product Chart 39

Appendix B List of Neem-Treated Conditions 47

Appendix C Planting a Neem Tree 53
    Why Plant a Neem Tree? 53
    Planting and Caring for Your Neem Tree 53
        Planting Your Neem Tree Outdoors 53
        Planting Your Neem Tree Indoors 54

Bibliography 55

About the Author 59

Index 61

Top 10 Facts About Neem

- Neem is anti–aging.

- Neem helps over 100 ailments.

- Neem has more antioxidants than blueberries.

- Neem has been used as medicine for thousands of years.

- Neem helps with dental hygiene, diabetes, and high blood pressure.

- Neem is used as a powerful anti–inflammatory, anti–cancer, and antibacterial agent.

- Neem is gentle and safe for people and pets.

- Neem can be used on nearly 500 pests.

- Neem can replace harmful pesticides.

- Neem is a soil enhancer and helps plants grow.

What People Are Saying About Neem

Andrew Weil, M.D. says neem is the botanical pesticide he uses most.

Dr. Oz Fans website: Neem bark extract is a "secret plaque fighter…neem extract acts as an anti–inflammatory and helps to prevent gum disease."

Dr. Bruce Jarvis, Professor Emeritus, University of Maryland: "Much of modern pharmacopeia as well as our agricultural resources can be traced back to indigenous plants that our ancestors first made use of thousands of years ago. Neem is a quintessential example of such a plant that even today has much to tell us about how nature works and how, with thoughtful scientific investigation, our lives can continue to be enriched by this marvelous ancient plant."

Honolulu Star Advertiser: "A long–term solution to a mosquito or insect problem would be to grow a neem tree."

Neem Author Ellen Norton: Neem is "curer of all ailments" in Sanskrit.

U.S. National Research Council: "To those millions in India neem has miraculous powers, and now scientists around the world are beginning to think they may be right…even some of the most cautious researchers are saying that 'neem deserves to be called a wonder plant.'"

Preface

Neem is a marvelous ancient plant with bountiful benefits for health and the environment. Even the greatest skeptics acknowledge how marvelous neem can be. This book explores the benefits of neem for health and the environment based on the scientific literature available.

Note to Reader

The information and advice provided in this book are not intended as a substitution for the advice of your physician or healthcare professionals. Consult your physician and healthcare professionals for all issues that may require medical attention or diagnosis, including before administering or undertaking any course of treatment or diet. Neither the author nor the publisher shall be liable or responsible for any loss or damage allegedly arising from any information or suggestion in this book, nor for websites or their content that are referred to in this book.

Acknowledgements

This book became possible because of some key people. Dr. Bruce Jarvis contributed copious amounts of time to the original neem scientific paper that is the foundation of this book. Robert Long supported me during the writing of this book and spent many hours editing the content. Congo Man Kemp gave me the support to keep going. Nick Miaoulis and Daphne de Gregory of Abaco Neem introduced to me to their farm as well as neem remedies that I have personally experienced to enhance my health. They as well as their staff I have come to know, Ellen Sands and Barbara Foreman, truly impressed upon me the necessity of believing in the work that you do.

Introduction

Neem has been used in traditional medicine for thousands of years. It is so much a part of traditional medicine that its translation from Sanskrit means "the curer of all ailments." And, indeed, there is a lot of truth in this translation.

Even in Western medicine, the reported medicinal benefits of neem are far-reaching, and include treatments for cancer, malaria, bacteria, fungus, parasites, skin diseases, and dental hygiene. In fact, the ailments neem treats are so diverse, it is hard to imagine where neem does not have a use.

In addition to health benefits, neem is also healthy for the environment. It is a soil enhancer and wards away nearly 500 species of pests.

With such a track record in place for thousands of years, it is easy to understand why neem is widely regarded as the "curer of all ailments."

This book provides information about neem for a general audience. For a technical discussion, refer to its complement book *Neem: Medicinal and Environmental Benefits* in the bibliography.

Introduction

Abaco Neem Story

2

Abaco Neem, on the island of Abaco in the Bahamas, is the only certified organic neem farm in the Bahamas and the entire Caribbean. It began in 1993 when Nick Miaoulis, a Bahamian, saw neem as a potential source of timber for boat and home building, since it was resistant to termites and worms.

As Miaoulis learned about neem's significant health benefits his vision became more personal and altruistic. Miaoulis became attracted to the plant's ability to help control high blood pressure and diabetes, two health problems common in his family and prevalent in the Bahamas.

Starting the Farm

Importing 8,000 seeds from India, and then beginning the farm, were the next steps in making the Abaco Neem dream reality. As a clothier he lacked experience in farming, but as a successful businessman Miaoulis recognized he needed to seek qualified help, and noted, "Surround yourself with good people and good things will come."

This is when Miaoulis approached Albert Albury, a long-time Abaco farmer. Albury, who was 70 years old at the time and had recently lost his wife of 50 years, had little interest. He doubted he would live long enough to see any neem trees bear fruit.

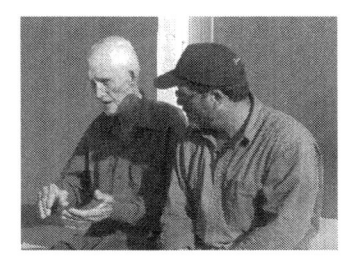

Albert Albury and Nick Miaoulis

Incidentally, Albury also had painful debilitating arthritis. At Miaoulis's urging, Albury began taking neem leaf in tea and encapsulated form for his arthritis, and his perspective on neem completely changed.

Albury began teaching Miaoulis about farming on Abaco and the seeds were started in a nursery. In 1994, Miaoulis acquired 120 acres (49 hectares) of land and established the Abaco Neem farm. Abaco Neem also began a nearby production center where the raw commodity from the farm is processed into a wide range of products. From this location they also manage their retail and wholesale distribution.

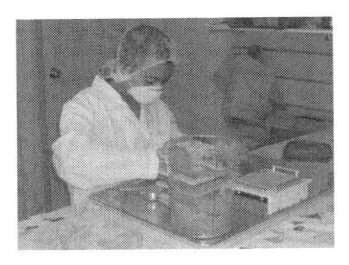

Abaco Neem Factory

Abaco Neem Farm Today

Today there are 6,200 neem trees on the Abaco Neem farm, along with a host of other trees and flowers—1,000 coconut trees, 3,000 aloe plants, citronella grass, and assorted citrus, tropical, flower, and berry trees. Of the over 200–acre (81–hectare) farm, 120 acres are cultivated.

The abundance of trees and flowers has provided a welcoming environment for birds and butterflies, attracting over 90 different species to the farm. Many other positive insect species are also present, including bee hives.

Today, Abaco Neem produces a range of products for the body, as well as pet and home and garden products. All of these are produced using organically grown neem.

Miaoulis said he is convinced he is providing the "best neem oil in the world." It would appear that others are inclined to agree, as Abaco Neem oil is considered "super high–grade quality neem oil" by the Neem Association and World Organization of Natural Medicine. His success resides in his farming methodology and the care in which he harvests.

The farm has a water table sufficient for neem growing conditions. Miaoulis enhances the soil quality with neem cake, seaweed, jumbey (wild tamarind) and ash. He then harvests neem fruit, leaves, and bark by hand: "All of our harvesting is done by hand on a daily basis, so only fresh ingredients are used to make products."

About the Neem Tree

Neem, a botanical cousin of mahogany, is native to Asia and Southeast Asia, and has since been transplanted to many parts of the world, including Africa, South America, Latin America, the Bahamas and other parts of the Caribbean, Middle East, and United States (AgroForestryTree Database).

Habitat—Dry, Hot, and Sunny

Except for waterlogged soil, neem can grow in almost any climate in the lowland tropics. Neem can grow within an altitude range of 0 to 5000 ft (0 to 1500 m), and tolerate conditions to 104°F (40°C) with a mean annual rainfall of 1.3 to 3.9 ft (400 to 1200 mm).

The adult neem is able to tolerate some frost, but requires a significant amount of sunlight. The young neem, on the other hand, can grow at least for the first few years in areas that are predominantly shaded, but is not able to tolerate frost (AgroForestryTree Database).

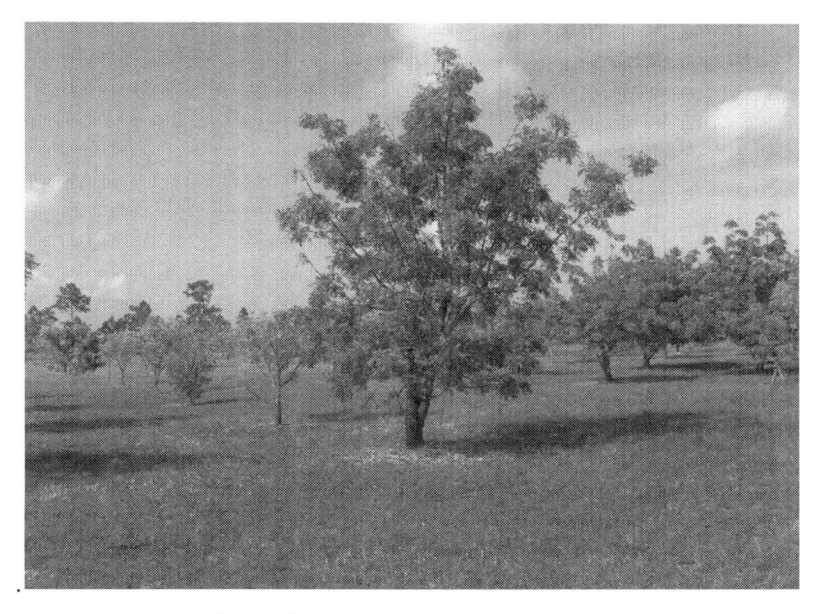

Neem Tree on the Abaco Neem Farm

About the Neem Tree

Neem can grow in soils from neutral to alkaline, but the optimum pH is 6.2 to 7. It can live well on shallow, stony, sandy soils, or where there is a hard calcareous or clay pan near the surface (AgroForestryTree Database). In an ideal habitat, neem can live 150 to 200 years (Neem Foundation).

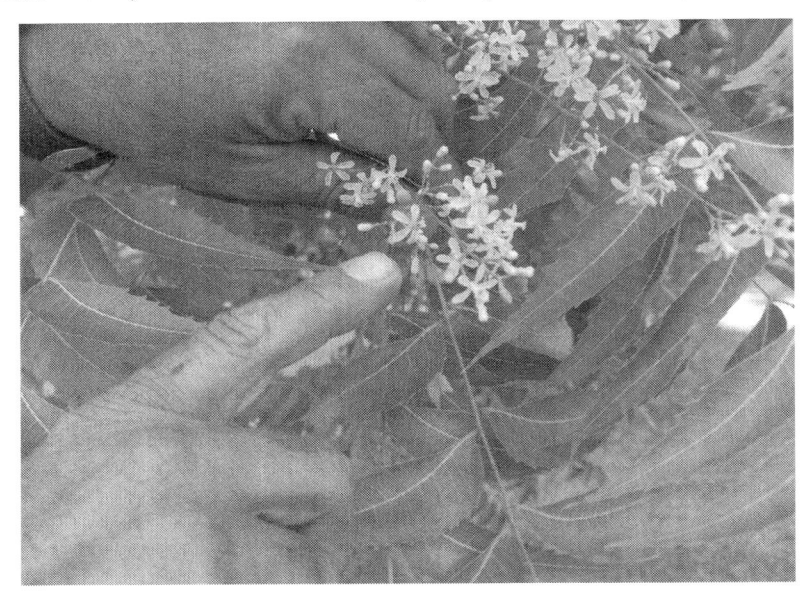

Neem Flowers

At four or five years old, neem can produce flowers and fruit, and after 10 to 12 years it will produce economically viable seed quantities (AgroForestryTree Database).

A mature tree produces 66 to 110 lb (30 to 50 kg) of fruit annually (Neem Foundation), or even as much as 220 lb (100 kg) of fruit per year (Cseke). It is pollinated by insects such as honeybees. The flowering and fruiting seasons vary, depending on the region and time of year (AgroForestryTree Database).

The fruit (about the size of an olive) is yellow when ripe, fleshy, and sweet with one (or perhaps two) seeds (Barceloux). It is eaten raw or cooked, and young twigs and flowers are sometimes eaten as vegetables. The fruit is also a major food source for birds and bats (they eat the pulp, not the seed), as well as other animals (AgroForestryTree Database).

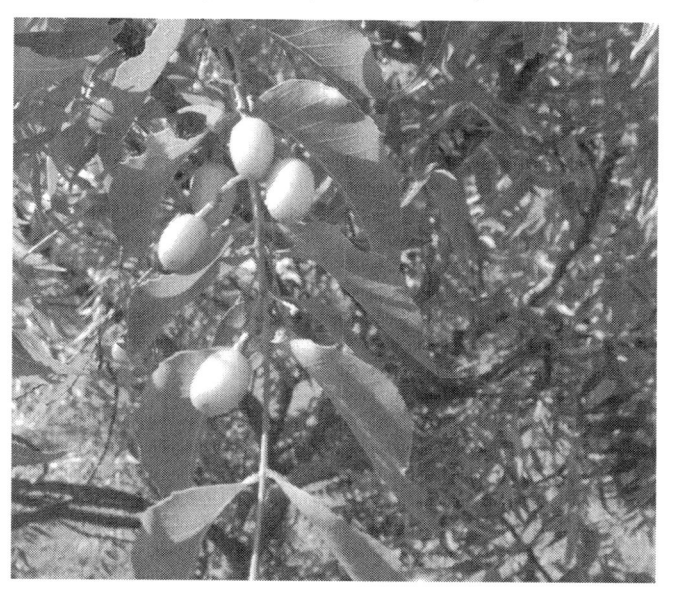

Neem Fruit

Chemistry of Neem

Neem is chemically rich and a pharmacy unto itself, with over 300 plant secondary compounds (Koul). Most of the active compounds are terpenoids, found in the fruit, seeds, twigs, stem, and root bark. Terpenoids provide plants aromatic qualities and are found in plants such as eucalyptus, cinnamon, cloves, and ginger.

Neem oil from the seed contains at least 35 pharmacologically active compounds (Cseke, Barceloux). Of all these chemicals, the main one that is used commercially is azadirachtin, which is unique to the neem tree.

Azadirachtin is a liminoid and, as the name suggests, is found in plants such as citrus. They stimulate detoxification as well as shrink tumors and inhibit their formation.

For an in–depth discussion of neem chemistry, refer to *Neem: Medicinal and Environmental Benefits* in the bibliography.

About the Neem Tree

Safety of Neem

Mitchell Fleisher, MD, DHt. DABFM, a double board–certified, homeopathic family physician and executive director of wellness of How2Connect.com, said he has treated hundreds of patients with purified neem extracts. In relation to the safety of neem, he said, "I have not observed a single, serious adverse reaction. Neem is clearly one of the safest—as well as most cost–effective—herbal medicines available today" (Sperber Haas, Fleisher).

The Neem Foundation reports that neem does not have any negative health effects for humans because it is gentle. In fact, the U.S. Environmental Protection Agency (EPA) acknowledges neem has been used "for millennia for medicinal, cosmetic, and pesticidal purposes…and adverse effects are not expected to humans, wildlife, or the environment."

In fact, neem has been found to be less toxic than table salt and aspirin in standard scientific tests. The LD50 value (Lethal Dose, 50%) indicates the amount of the substance needed to kill half of the test subjects. Where a 150 lb (68 kg) human would only need to ingest 2.8 oz (0.082 L) of aspirin and 8.0 oz (0.237 L) of table salt to reach that lethal dosage, those same test subjects would need to ingest 18 oz (.532 L) of neem in order to reach the lethal dose (Sperber Haas).

While many parts of the neem tree can be ingested internally (that is, leaves, bark, and fruit), neem oil is not recommended to be ingested internally and is not approved by the FDA for internal human use. Neem oil is safe to apply topically.

Caution: Always consult your medical practitioner before taking any new medication, including neem.

Remedies by Health Topic   5

Dr. Fleisher said he has treated hundreds of patients with purified neem extracts. Dr. Fleisher stated that he has successfully prescribed neem for a broad range of health issues, including dental abscesses, pneumonia, inflammatory bowel disease, acne, asthma, rheumatoid arthritis, psoriasis, sinusitis, lice, scabies, and serious bacterial, viral, fungal or parasitic infections (Sperber Haas, Fleisher).

Dr. Fleisher said neem possesses "powerful anti–inflammatory, as well as broad spectrum antiviral, antibacterial, antifungal, antiparasitic and anti–neoplastic properties that, in certain individuals, may help eliminate infections, prevent formation of abnormal cells, and accelerate healing" (Sperber Haas, Fleisher).

List of Neem Remedies by Health Topic

Below is the list of common uses for neem as well as the Abaco Neem product that may be used for treatment. More information is available in Appendix B and at www.abaconeem.com.

Acne

Daily Moisturizer

Neem Cream

Neem Leaf Capsules (for detoxification and cleansing)

Neem Soap (assorted)

Anti–bacterial

First Aid Spray

Neem Leaf Capsules

Neem Leaf Extract

Neem Oil

Neem Soap (assorted)

Antifungal

First Aid Spray

Neem Leaf Extract

Neem Oil

Neem Soap (assorted)

Antiseptic
First Aid Spray
Neem Leaf Extract

Arthritic pain
Neem Leaf Tea and/or Neem Leaf Capsules
Neem Salve

Asthma
Neem Leaf Capsules (for long–term prevention)
Neem Leaf Extract (for immediate response)

Athlete's foot
First Aid Spray
Neem Leaf Extract
Neem Salve
Neem Soap (assorted)

Bowel movement regulation
Neem Leaf Capsules
Neem Leaf Tea

Burns
Neem Leaf Capsules (open capsule and apply powder)
Neem Oil
Neem Salve

Chicken pox
Neem Leaf Tea (to bathe skin)
Neem Lotion
Neem Salve or Neem Oil
Neem Soap (assorted)

Cold sores
Lip Balm
Neem Leaf Capsules (for internal detoxification)

Neem Leaf Extract or First Aid Spray
Neem Salve

Dandruff
Neem Hair and Scalp Conditioner
Neem Oil
Neem Shampoo Body Wash

Dental hygiene
Neem Bark Tooth Powder
Neem Leaf Extract

Diabetes
Neem Leaf Capsules
Neem Leaf Extract
Neem Leaf Tea
Neem Salve

Diaper rash
Neem & Aloe Body Lotion
Neem Salve
Neem Soap (oatmeal or coconut almond)

Earache
Neem Leaf Extract

Eczema
Neem & Aloe Body Lotion
Neem Cream
Neem Leaf Capsules
Neem Oil
Neem Salve
Neem Soap (assorted)

Gingivitis
First Aid Spray
Neem Bark Tooth Powder
Neem Leaf Extract

Remedies by Health Topic

Gum disease
　Neem Bark Tooth Powder
　Neem Leaf Extract
　Neem Oil

Gums, bleeding
　Neem Bark Tooth Powder
　Neem Leaf Extract

Hair moisturizer
　Neem Hair & Scalp Conditioner
　Neem Oil
　Neem Shampoo Body Wash

High blood pressure
　Neem Leaf Capsules
　Neem Leaf Tea

Immune system
　Neem Leaf Capsules
　Neem Leaf Tea
　Neem Oil

Inflammation
　Neem Leaf Capsules
　Neem Oil
　Neem Salve

Insomnia
　Neem Leaf Capsules
　Neem Leaf Tea

Joint pain
　Neem Leaf Capsules
　Neem Salve

Lice
　First Aid Spray
　Neem Oil

Neem Shampoo Body Wash

Lips, chapped
Lip balm

Mosquitoes
First Aid Spray
Neem and Citronella Candles
Neem Insect Repellent

Muscle pain
Neem Leaf Capsules
Neem Salve

Pest repellent
Neem and Citronella Candles
Neem Insect Repellent

Psoriasis
Neem & Aloe Body Lotion
Neem Oil
Neem Salve
Neem Soap (assorted)

Ringworm
First Aid Spray
Neem Leaf Extract
Neem Shampoo Body Wash

Sand flies (noseeums)
Neem and Citronella Candles
Neem Insect Repellent

Scalp (seborrheic dermatitis)
Neem Oil
Neem Shampoo Body Wash

Scalp, dry and flaky
Neem Hair & Scalp Conditioner

Neem Oil
Neem Shampoo Body Wash

Scar tissue (keloids)
Neem Oil

Scars
Neem Oil
Neem Salve

Serotonin increaser
Neem Leaf Capsules
Neem Leaf Tea

Skin age spots
Daily Moisturizer
Neem Cream
Neem Oil

Skin, anti-aging
Daily Moisturizer
Neem Cream
Neem Oil

Skin cancers
Daily Moisturizer
Neem & Aloe Body Lotion
Neem Oil

Skin conditions
Neem & Aloe Body Lotion
Neem Oil
Neem Shampoo Body Wash
Neem Soap (assorted)

Skin discoloration
Daily Moisturizer
Neem & Aloe Body Lotion

List of Neem Remedies by Health Topic

    Neem Balm (assorted)
    Neem Cream
    Neem Soap (assorted)

Skin elasticity
    Daily Moisturizer
    Neem & Aloe Body Lotion
    Neem Cream
    Neem Oil
    Neem Salve

Skin moisturizer
    Daily Moisturizer
    Neem & Aloe Body Lotion
    Neem Balm (assorted)
    Neem Cream
    Neem Oil

Skin rashes
    Neem & Aloe Body Lotion
    Neem Leaf Tea (in a bath soak)
    Neem Salve or Neem Oil
    Neem Soap (assorted)

Skin, dry
    Daily Moisturizer or Neem & Aloe Body Lotion
    Neem Oil
    Neem Salve
    Neem Shampoo Body Wash
    Neem Soap (assorted)

Skin, itchy or irritated
    Daily Moisturizer
    Neem Aloe and Body Lotion
    Neem Balm
    Neem Cream

Neem Salve
Neem Shampoo Body Wash
Neem Soap (assorted)

Skin, preventing irritation and bumps
First Aid Spray
Neem & Aloe Body Lotion
Neem Balm
Neem Salve
Neem Shampoo Body Wash
Neem Soap (assorted)

Skin, sensitive and easily irritated
Daily Moisturizer
Neem & Aloe Body Lotion
Neem Balm (assorted)
Neem Shampoo Body Wash
Neem Soap (assorted)

Sore throat
First Aid Spray
Neem Leaf Extract

Stress
Neem Leaf Capsules

Stretch marks
Neem Oil
Neem Salve

Sunburns
Daily Moisturizer
Neem & Aloe Body Lotion
Neem Cream

Toothache
Neem Bark Tooth Powder
Neem Leaf Extract

Wound healing
First Aid Spray

Neem Leaf Capsules (open capsule and apply powder)

Neem Oil

Neem Salve

Remedies by Health Topic

Select Health Issues 6

This section contains information from scientific studies about the efficacy of neem for medicinal applications. It is provided for those readers who are interested in the scientific literature. For more information about this technical discussion, refer to *Neem: Medicinal and Environmental Benefits* in the bibliography.

Chemical Complexity of Neem

Neem has been used as a medicinal agent for thousands of years. In traditional medicine, all parts of the neem tree are used—flowers, seeds, fruits, roots, bark, and in particular, leaves—to treat more than 100 diseases (Neem Foundation). Despite thousands of years of use, neem (like other botanicals) is so complex the mode of action for neem chemicals is not clearly understood nor described in published studies. Azadirachtin itself is so chemically complex its structure was not determined conclusively until 1987, and it was not synthesized in the lab until 20 years later by Dr. Steve Ley and 40 PhD students (Veitch and Devakumar).

For many reasons, including its chemical complexity (as discussed in *Neem: Medicinal and Environmental Benefits*), neem has not yet been approved for internal use by the United States Federal Drug Administration. Despite this absence of approval, neem has many high-profile supporters in the U.S. medical community, including Dr. Mehmet Oz. He touted neem bark extract as the "secret plaque fighter...neem extract acts as an anti-inflammatory and helps to prevent gum disease."

Antioxidant

Antioxidants are known to have a role in preventing degenerative cell damage that can lead to diseases such as atherosclerosis, diabetes, and heart disease. All forms of neem have been found to be extremely high in antioxidants, far higher than popular antioxidant foods such as blueberries, broccoli, and cranberries, as shown in the Oxygen Radical Absorbance Capacity (ORAC) test (Sperber Haas):

Item	ORAC Per Gram
Tomatoes	4.60
Grapefruit	15.48
Broccoli	15.90

Item	ORAC Per Gram
Spinach	26.40
Blueberries	62.20
Plums	62.39
Cranberry	94.56
Neem/supercritical extract (8% in sesame oil)	114.00
Neem leaf	**357.00**
Neem oil	**430.06**
Neem bark	**476.00**

Cancer

A number of neem chemicals have been shown to be active in several cancer studies, including prostate, colon, and breast. In addition, neem leaf has been found to be active in inducing apoptosis in tumor cells (programmed cell death, causing the cancer cells to rupture), and in enhancing an antigen associated with breast tumor in mice and rats. In addition, a chemical from neem flowers, nimbolide, was shown to restrict cancer cell proliferation (Kumar, Roy, Bose, Mandal–Ghosh).

While neem has shown a lot of promise in battling cancer, it is not recommended as a replacement for conventional cancer therapies.

Dental and Oral Care

Neem has benefits in dental and oral care by inhibiting bacteria that causes tooth decay. In preliminary findings, neem inhibited *Streptococcus mutans* (bacterium causing tooth decay) and reversed incipient carious lesions (that is, primary dental caries) (Vanka).

When saliva–conditioned hydroxyapatite (a bone salt that strengthens the matrix of teeth and bone) was pre–treated with neem extract (from bark sticks) there was major inhibition in some Streptococcus colonization on tooth surfaces (Wolinsky). As mango is also known to inhibit other microorganisms that cause dental caries (*Streptococcus mutans*, *Streptococcus salivarius*, *Streptococcus mitis*, and *Streptococcus sanguis*), chewing both mango and neem tree sticks would provide even further benefit (Prashant).

Furthermore, a neem–extract dental gel significantly reduced plaque and bacteria (*Streptococcus mutans* and *Lactobacilli* species were tested) over the control group that used commercially available mouthwash containing the germicide chlorhexidine gluconate (0.2% w/v) (Pai).

Diabetes

Neem significantly reduced diabetic symptoms in non–insulin dependent diabetics. These symptoms included polydypsia (excessive thirst), polyuria (increased frequency of urination), polyphagia (excessive hunger) and fatigue, and less commonly sweating, burning feet, itching, and headaches (Kochhar). Studies have also found that using neem can help reduce the need for insulin, and possibly prevent or delay the onset of diabetes (Sperber Haas).

HIV/AIDS

Neem has been found to be useful in HIV/AIDS treatments. An oral administration of acetone–water neem leaf extract had a "significant" influence on cells HIV affects, and is recommended as part of an HIV/AIDS drug treatment program (Mbah).

Pregnancy and Contraception

While there are no neem pregnancy and contraception products available in the United States, a product in India has shown promise in clinical trials to be effective in immobilizing sperm (Joshi, Garg).

In addition, a fraction of neem oil has been found to have antifertility, anti–implantation, and abortifacient properties, which makes it a "highly desirable potential vaginal contraceptive agent" (Sharma).

Furthermore, neem and seed extracts administered orally at the beginning of the post–implantation stage resulted in pregnancy termination in rodents and primates, without any permanent effects (Talwar).

Skin Disorders

Neem can treat many skin disorders, including scabies and lice.

In a paste combination with turmeric, neem was used to treat scabies in 814 people—97% of them were cured within 3 to 15 days of application, with no adverse reactions observed (Charles).

Also, a new formulation of neem shampoo has proven to be "highly effective against all stages of head lice" even after only 10 minutes of exposure time. The percentages of effectiveness ranged from 86% to 97% after a single application of the shampoo. Only two retreatments were needed for most children to remain lice–free. No adverse effects were observed (Abdel–Ghaffar).

Ulcers

Neem bark extract reduced human gastric acid hypersecretion, and gastroesophageal and gastroduodenal ulcers. After 10 weeks, the duodenal ulcers were nearly fully healed. After just six weeks, one case of esophageal ulcer and gastric ulcer was fully healed (Bandyopadhyay).

Pet Health Benefits

Neem holds many benefits for the four–legged members of the family. Abaco Neem recommends the following treatments for pets:

Neem Oil

A highly potent antimicrobial that disinfects while healing cuts, scrapes, and other skin breakages as well as warts. Neem is a natural repellent against hundreds of insects and pests including fleas, ticks and mosquitoes. Studies have shown that neem oil is effective in shrinking cancer tumors. Apply directly onto the skin.

Pet Shampoo

Non–irritating and containing neem oil, the pet shampoo is a very effective repellent against fleas and ticks and is soothing to irritated skin disorders. Allow shampoo to stay on skin at least three to five minutes before rinsing.

Pet Caps

A natural immune stimulant and dewormer, pet caps provide protection against skin disorders, enhance circulation, and reduce inflammation which is particularly beneficial for arthritis.

Pet Salve

Effective as a topical anti–inflammatory for arthritic joint pain and skin issues. Apply to hot spots and skin, such as the underside of paws.

Neem Leaf Extract

Neem, being antiviral and antibacterial, is a natural treatment for sore throat and gums, earache, or wherever there is threat of bacterial infection, such as bites or cuts. Apply two drops in the ear twice daily and/or ¼ dropper in the throat. To avoid contamination, be careful not to let the dropper touch your pet.

Neem Trees and Leaves

Very effective repellent against fleas, ticks, cockroaches, mosquitoes, termites, and many other insects and pests. Planting trees around kennels and in areas where pets live provide both cooling shade and protection from insects and pests. The leaves can be spread on the ground around and under kennels. Leaves if eaten by pets are also beneficial to them.

Pet Health Benefits

Neem Seed Cake

The remaining part of the seed after oil has been pressed from it, neem seed cake still contains a considerable amount of oil. It can be soaked for six to eight hours in water and used as a dip or spray on pets or kennel. Use ½ cup (0.114 L) of neem seed cake for a 5 gallon (19 L) container.

Remedies by Pet Health Topic

Below is the list of neem uses for your pet as well as the neem product that may be used for treatment. For more information, visit www.abaconeem.com.

Health Topic	Recommended Product
Arthritic pain	Neem Pet Capsules
	Neem Pet Salve
Dewormer	Neem Pet Capsules
Ear Mites	Neem Leaf Extract
Fleas	Neem Pet Shampoo
Fur, healthy	Neem Pet shampoo
Hot spots	Neem Pet Salve
Immune system	Neem Pet Capsules
Joint inflammation	Neem Pet Capsule
	Neem Pet Salve
Joint pain	Neem Pet Capsules
	Neem Pet Salve
Mange	Neem Pet Shampoo
	Neem Pet Salve
Parasites	Neem Pet Capsules
Paws, damaged	Neem Pet Salve
Skin health	Neem Pet Shampoo
Ticks	Neem Pet Shampoo

Enviro- and Agri-Benefits   8

While some plants are known to be invasive species and negative for their environment, neem appears to be only positive for its environment, no matter where it is planted. Neem is known to:

- Put more nutrients into the soil than it takes out
- Need very little rain
- Be wind and salt tolerant
- Maintain and restore soil fertility
- Keep the environment clean and cool the air space

Erosion Control

Neem has a well-developed root system that can extract nutrients from lower soil levels. This aspect of neem makes it an important agent in erosion control because it is virtually drought-resistant. As such, it is useful as a dune fixation tree (AgroForestryTree Database).

Soil Enhancer

Farmers use neem cake as an organic manure and soil amendment. Neem cake enhances the efficiency of nitrogen fertilizers by reducing the rate of nitrification and hampering pests such as nematodes, fungi, and insects (AgroForestryTree Database).

Parasite Control

The Abaco Big Bird chicken farm, a 93-acre (38-hectare) chicken farm in the Bahamas, used neem cake to help control the deadly parasite cocci, which attacks digestive tracts of young chickens, costing the global chicken industry billions of dollars annually.

Representative Lance Pinder reported that chicken health noticeably improved after neem was introduced into the diet, staving off cocci, which Pinder said is the biggest challenge to any commercial chicken farm. Abaco Big Bird also reported equal or better conversion ratios (a measure of how much feed it takes to grow a pound of chicken) over conventional therapies since using neem. Chicks have improved survival rates, no longer need vaccination, and have a noticeably healthier look in their physical appearance.

Pesticide—Gentle and Safe

Neem is active as a pesticide in nearly 500 species of pests mostly due to azadirachtin which is known as the "most potent insect antifeedant discovered to date" (Ishaaya). Pests include beetles, weevils, cockroaches, aphids, termites, grasshoppers, thrips, and fleas. Abaco Neem reports that their pet shampoo is very effective at repelling fleas.

Azadirachtin may affect insects in the following ways (Anuradha, Mordue, Koul):

- Antifeedant: causes anorexia
- Insect growth regulation: reduced growth, increased mortality, abnormal and delayed molts
- Sterility/reproduction: reduced number of viable eggs and live progeny, affects sperm formation
- Cellular processes: blocks cell division in meiosis and mitosis
- Muscles: causes loss of muscle tone
- Cell synthetic machinery: blocks digestive enzyme production in gut, and inhibits protein synthesis.

Along with insects, neem has also been suggested as an effective infertility agent in controlling populations of rodents, such as rats (Morovati). It may also be useful in controlling foodborne pathogens, making it a potential agent against food spoilage bacteria (Hoque). Neem has also been cited as effective against a goldfish pathogen (*Aeromonas hydrophila*) that causes significant losses to fisheries (Harikrishnan). By far, though, the most common use of neem is against insects.

While many insects feed on neem, neem has very few serious pests of its own. Approximately 35 known pests feed on its sap, bark, roots, shoots, and leaves. These pests include shoot borers, termites (*Microtermes)*, fungus (*Psuedocercospora subsesessilis*), mistletoes (*Dendrophtoe falcate, Tapinanthus* spp), and bacteria (*Pseudomonas azadirachtae*) (AgroForestryTree Database, Cseke). Two serious pests to neem are the scale insect (*Aonidiella orientalis)*, and the tea mosquito bug *(Helopeltis antonii)*.

Citrus Tree Pest Reduction

Neem has been found to significantly reduce pests on a citrus farm. Farmer Jerry Newton reported positive effects of neem towards reducing pests such as rust mites and beetles, as well as a sooty mold that was affecting crop yield and growth. In the 1990s he applied a neem leaf–water mixture to his

200–acre (81 hectare) farm of citrus fruits. After one week, he noticed less sooty mold on the trees, and a significant reduction of rust mites. He was forced to cease his experiment due to hurricanes, but a year later he revisited the use of neem with a new organic pesticide business. He applied a neem cake–water mixture on citrus trees and after two weeks observed the same results as with the citrus farm. "Patience with neem is the key," Newton said. Neem will not "knock 'em dead" with the first spray, but over three months the numbers of pests were "dramatically reduced."

A Future with Less Harmful Pesticides?

Neem has little if any effect on most beneficial pests, such as spiders, lady beetles, parasitic wasps, and predatory mites, nor does it affect levels of honey bee pollinations or worker bees (Hall). Azadirachtin is also not toxic to birds or bees but may be to some fish, according to the University of Delaware.

Neem by most accounts offers a promising future as a mosquito repellent (Vatandoost), and can be a "very useful" component of an integrated approach against malaria transmission because of its efficacy, low cost, and safety, especially when compared to synthetic insecticides (Gianotti).

Since neem does not kill adult insects, neem–based insecticides tend to be used with other strategies like adulticides (to kill adult insects) or beneficial pests (Hall). Considering that synthetic insecticides are more dangerous, leave toxic residues in food, are not readily biodegradable (Peshin), and can harm beneficial pests, neem offers a sound alternative in these respects, even though it is not as powerful as synthetic agents such as permethrin and DEET (which may be a consideration for areas at high–risk for malaria).

Using Neem as a Pesticide in Your Home

Neem has been used successfully as a home pesticide for thousands of years. It is as easy as mixing neem oil with water, and then adding a bit of soap or natural emulsifier to keep the oil and water mixed. Use between 1 tablespoon and to 1 ounce (0.03 L) of oil per gallon of water, and then add some soap to mix the oil and water. Use within 24 hours for optimum results (Sperber Haas). Abaco Neem has created a full range of commercial and home use agricultural products.

Enviro- and Agri-Benefits

Learning More   9

Nick Miaoulis, founder of the Abaco Neem farm, said he is a strong advocate of the benefits of neem, in particular how neem can be used to promote health and pesticide–free agriculture: "I am committed to doing everything I can to promote and encourage the protection of our valuable water and environment."

Abaco Neem staff provide guided tours of the farm to schools, researchers, and others interested in learning about the wonders of neem. Staff at the farm and factory are also helpful in providing guidance about neem in general.

Learning More

Appendix A Product Chart

Below is a list of Abaco Neem products and how they may be used to assist with various health issues. More information is available on www.abaconeem.com.

Daily Moisturizer

Acne

Skin age spots

Skin cancer

Skin discoloration

Skin, dry

Skin elasticity

Skin, anti–ageing

Skin moisturizer

Skin, itchy or irritated

Skin, sensitive and easily irritated

Sunburns

First Aid Spray

Anti–bacterial

Antifungal

Antiseptic

Athlete's foot

Cold sores

Gingivitis

Lice

Mosquitoes

Ringworm

Skin, preventing irritation and bumps

Sore throat

Wound healing

Lip Balm
   Cold sores
   Lips, chapped

Neem & Aloe Body Lotion
   Diaper rash
   Eczema
   Psoriasis
   Skin cancers
   Skin conditions
   Skin discoloration
   Skin elasticity
   Skin, itchy or irritated
   Skin moisturizer
   Skin, preventing irritation and bumps
   Skin rashes
   Skin, dry
   Skin, sensitive and easily irritated
   Sunburns

Neem and Citronella Candles
   Mosquitoes
   Pest repellent
   Sand flies (noseeums)

Neem Balm
   Skin discoloration
   Skin moisturizer
   Skin, itchy or irritated
   Skin, preventing irritation and bumps
   Skin, sensitive and easily irritated

Neem Bark Tooth Powder
   Dental hygiene
   Gingivitis

Gum disease
Gums, bleeding
Toothache

Neem Hair & Scalp Conditioner
Dandruff
Hair moisturizer
Scalp, dry and flaky

Neem Cream
Acne
Eczema
Skin age spots
Skin, anti–ageing
Skin discoloration
Skin elasticity
Skin, itchy or irritated
Skin moisturizer
Sunburns

Neem Insect Repellent
Mosquitoes
Pest repellent
Sand flies (noseeums)

Neem Leaf Capsules
Acne
Anti–bacterial
Arthritic pain
Asthma
Bowel movement regulation
Burns
Cold sores
Diabetes
Eczema

    High blood pressure
    Immune system
    Inflammation
    Insomnia
    Joint pain
    Muscle pain
    Serotonin increaser
    Stress
    Wound healing

Neem Leaf Extract
    Anti–bacterial
    Antifungal
    Antiseptic
    Asthma
    Athlete's foot
    Cold sores
    Dental hygiene
    Diabetes
    Earache
    Gingivitis
    Gum disease
    Gums, bleeding
    Ring worm
    Sore throat
    Toothache

Neem Leaf Tea
    Arthritic pain
    Bowel movement regulation
    Chicken pox
    Diabetes
    High blood pressure

Immune system
Insomnia
Serotonin raiser
Skin rashes (as a bath soak)

Neem Lotion
Chicken pox

Neem Oil
Anti–bacterial
Antifungal
Burns
Chicken pox
Dandruff
Eczema
Gum disease
Hair moisturizer
Immune system
Inflammation
Lice
Psoriasis
Scalp (seborrheic dermatitis)
Scalp, dry and flaky
Scar tissue (keyloyds)
Scars
Skin age spots
Skin rashes
Skin, anti–ageing
Skin cancers
Skin conditions
Skin, dry
Skin elasticity
Skin moisturizer

Stretch marks
Wound healing

Neem Salve
Arthritic pain
Athlete's foot
Burns
Chicken pox
Cold sores
Diabetes
Diaper rash
Eczema
Inflammation
Joint pain
Muscle pain
Psoriasis
Scars
Skin elasticity
Skin, itchy or irritated
Skin, preventing irritation and bumps
Skin rashes
Skin, dry
Stretch marks
Wound healing

Neem Shampoo Body Wash
Dandruff
Hair moisturizer
Lice
Ring worm
Scalp (seborrheic dermatitis)
Scalp, dry and flaky
Skin conditions

Skin, dry

Skin, itchy or irritated

Skin, preventing irritation and bumps

Skin, sensitive and easily irritated

Neem Soap (assorted)

Acne

Anti–bacterial

Antifungal

Athlete's foot

Chicken pox

Diaper rash

Eczema

Psoriasis

Skin conditions

Skin discoloration

Skin, dry

Skin rashes

Skin, itchy or irritated

Skin, preventing irritation and bumps

Skin, sensitive and easily irritated

Appendix B List of Neem-Treated Conditions

As more research is conducted, the list of conditions neem treats just gets longer. The list below represents all the neem-treated conditions verified through scientific research at the time of printing. This impressive list demonstrates neem to be the ultimate health herb:

A

Abortifacient

Acne

Anti-anxiety

Antibacterial

Anticarcinogenic

Anticlotting

Anticomplement (similar to antioxidant)

Antifeedant

Antifertility

Antifungal

Anti-gastric (ulcer)

Antihepatic

Antihistamine

Antihyperglycemic

Anti-implantation

Anti-inflammatory

Antileprosy

Antimalarial

Antimicrobial

Antimutagenic

Antioxidant

Antiparasitic

Antiperiodic
Antiperiodontic
Antipurgative
Anti–pyretic (fever)
Antirheumatic
Antiseptic
Antituberculosis
Antitumor
Antiulcer
Antiviral
Antiworm
Arthritic pain
Asthma
Athlete's foot

B
Bacterial infection
Blood detoxifier
Boils
Bowel movement regulation
Burns

C
Chicken pox
Cold sores

D
Dandruff
Dental hygiene
Diabetes
Diaper rash
Diuretic

E
Earache

Eczema
Eye diseases

F

Fungal infection

G

Gingivitis
Gum disease
Gums, bleeding

H

Hair moisturizer
High blood pressure
HIV/AIDS

I

Immune system
Immunomodulatory
Inflammation
Inflammatory bowel disease
Insomnia

J

Joint pain

L

Lice
Lips, chapped

M

Mosquitoes
Muscle pain

P

Parasitic infection
Pest repellent
Pimples

Pneumonia

Psoriasis

R

Ringworm

S

Sand flies (noseeums)

Scabies

Scalp (seborrheic dermatitis)

Scalp, dry and flaky

Scars

Scar tissue (keyloyds)

Serotonin raiser

Sinusitis

Skin age spots

Skin cancers

Skin conditions

Skin discoloration

Skin diseases

Skin elasticity

Skin moisturizer

Skin rashes

Skin, anti–ageing

Skin, dry

Skin, itchy or irritated

Skin, preventing irritation and bumps

Skin, sensitive and easily irritated

Sore throat

Spermicidal

Stretch marks

Sunburns

T

Toothache

V

Viral infections

W

Wound healing

Source: AgroForestryTree Database, Cseke, Subapriya, Boeke, Talwar, Liu, Conrick.

Appendix C Planting a Neem Tree

Neem is a very hardy tree and does not require very much maintenance. Abaco Neem has helped many people plant their own neem trees, including customers, schools, businesses, and community organizations.

Why Plant a Neem Tree?

Traditionally neem trees have been planted near homes to ward away mosquitos and insects. The Honolulu Star Advertiser reported that "A long-term solution to a mosquito or insect problem would be to grow a neem tree."

There are other reasons to plant neem trees in your environment. The neem tree prevents soil erosion. It is also useful as an environmentally friendly organic manure and soil amendment, as well as a nitrogen fertilizer enhancer.

Even the neem leaves are useful to your environment. The leaves can be placed around trees and homes, and in cupboards, drawers and attics to deter roaches, termites, and other insects.

Planting and Caring for Your Neem Tree

Neem is a very hardy tree. Except for waterlogged soil, neem can grow in almost any climate in the lowland tropics, including the Caribbean and United States.

Planting Your Neem Tree Outdoors

Abaco Neem provides the following guidelines for planting your neem tree:

1. Dig a hole twice as deep and twice as wide as the pot that your tree is in. Fill the hole with good draining soil, add water to wet the soil, and then plant the tree only as deep as it was in the original pot (that is, roots only).
2. Water again after stepping down the soil around tree to eliminate any air pockets that may be in the soil.
3. Water every couple of days until the tree is established. Then, water only as needed, as indicated when the leaves droop.

4. When the tree is about three to four feet high (1 to 1.2 m) from the soil level, prune back about one foot (0.3 m) at a 45° angle. Look for indications of new shoots growing and prune just above them.

Note: Do not plant your neem tree where there is a threat of water settling as the root system cannot handle very much water. The tree only needs about 18 inches (.5 m) of rain a year and is quite drought–resistant.

5. After pruning, you will soon see two to three new branches growing. When these branches are about two to three feet (0.6 to 0.9 m) long, you can prune them in the same way as above. Continue pruning each year to your desired size. For best protection against strong weather, do not allow the tree to grow higher than 30 to 40 feet (9 to 12 m).

6. If you have additional trees, plant them about 20 feet (6 m) apart to allow for full growth.

Planting Your Neem Tree Indoors

When planting your neem tree indoors, follow these guidelines (Sperber Haas):

- Plant your tree in the largest pot you have (they will not grow larger than their pots).
- Use soil specifically designated for houseplants.
- After you plant the neem tree in the pot, water thoroughly and then do not water again until the leaves become droopy.
- Initially, do not overexpose a young tree to sun (avoid afternoon sun). As the tree grows it will benefit from being placed in a location where it experiences full sun.
- Your neem tree may be fertilized on a monthly basis if desired, using a balanced organic fertilizer such as 6–6–6.
- Should you want to harvest neem year round, be sure to continue to expose your neem tree to light even in the winter months. Shine a general living room lamp on your neem tree for several hours in the evening.

Note: If you are starting your neem tree from a seed, obtain specific instructions for growing from the nursery.

Bibliography

Abaco Neem Farm fact sheets and interviews, 2009–2112.

Abdel–Ghaffar F, Semmler M. Efficacy of neem seed extract shampoo on head lice of naturally infected humans in Egypt. *Parasitol Res.* 2007, 100(2):329–32.

Anuradha A, Annadurai RS. Biochemical and molecular evidence of azadirachtin binding to insect actins. *Current Science.* 2008, 95(11).

Azadirachta indica. AgroForestryTree Database website. Accessed March 16, 2009.

Bandyopadhyay U, Biswas K, Sengupta A, Moitra P, Dutta P, Sarkar D, Debnath P, Ganguly CK, Banerjee RK. Clinical studies on the effect of Neem (Azadirachta indica) bark extract on gastric secretion and gastroduodenal ulcer. *Life Sci.* 2004, 75:2867–2878.

Barceloux, D. *Medical Toxicology of Natural Substances.* John Wiley & Sons, Inc. 2008.

Boeke SJ, Boersma MG, Alink GM, van Loon JJ, van Huis A, Dicke M, Rietjens IM. Safety evaluation of Neem (Azadirachta indica) derived pesticides. *J Ethnopharmacol.* 2004, 94(1):25–41.

Bose A, Haque E, Baral R. Neem leaf preparation induces apoptosis of tumor cells by releasing cytotoxic cytokines from human peripheral blood mononuclear cells. *Phytother Res.* 2007, 21(10):914–20.

Charles V, Charles SX. The use and efficacy of Azadirachta indica ADR (neem) and Curcuma longa (turmeric) in scabies. A pilot study. *Trop Geogr Med.* 1992, 44(1–2):178–81.

Conrick, John. *Neem the Ultimate Herb.* Lotus Press. 2009.

Cseke LJ, Kirakosyan A, Kaufman PB, Warber SL, Duke J, Brielmann HL. *Natural Products from Plants, 2nd edition.* Taylor & Francis Group. 2006.

De Gregory, Daphne. Sales and marketing representative of Abaco Neem. Personal interviews. 2009–2012.

Devakumar C, Kumar R. Total synthesis of azadirachtin: A chemical odyssey. *Current Science.* 2008, 95(5).

"Dr. Oz: vitamin E Causes Cancer, Neem Bark Extract and Gum Disease." Dr. Oz Fans website. Accessed May 22, 2011.

Environmental Protection Agency website.

Fleisher, Mitchell, MD, DHt., DABFM, DcABCT. Email correspondence. January 21, 2011.

Bibliography

Garg S, Doncel G, Chabra S, Upadhyay SN, Talwar GP. Synergistic spermicidal activity of Neem seed extract, reetha saponins and quinine hydrochloride. *Contraception.* 1994, 50(2):185–90.

Gianotti RL, Bomblies A, Dafalla M, Issa–Arzika I, Duchemin JB, Eltahir EA. Efficacy of local neem extracts for sustainable malaria vector control in an African village. *Malar J.* 2008 7:138.

Hall FR, Menn JJ, editors. *Biopesticides Use and Delivery.* Humana Press. 1999.

Harikrishnan R, Balasundaram C. In vitro and in vivo studies of the use of some medicinal herbals against the pathogen Aeromonas hydrophila in goldfish. *J Aquat Anim Health.* 2008, 20(3):165–76.

Hoque M, Bari ML, Inatsu Y, Juneja VK, Kawamoto S. Antibacterial activity of guava (Psidium guajava L.) and neem (Azadirachta indica A. Juss.) extracts against foodborne pathogens and spoilage bacteria. *Foodborne Pathog Dis.* 2007, 4(4):481–8.

Ishaaya I, Nauen R, Horowitz AR, editors. *Insecticides Design Using Advanced Technologies.* Springer–Verlag. 2007.

Joshi SN, Dutta S, Kumar BK, Katti U, Kulkarni S, Risbud A, Mehendale S. Expanded safety study of Praneem polyherbal vaginal tablet among HIV–uninfected women in Pune, India: a phase II clinical trial report. *Sexually Transmitted Infections.* 2008, 84:343–347.

Kochhar A, Sharma N, Sachdeva R. Effect of supplementation of tulsi (Ocimum sanctum) and neem (Azadirachta indica) leaf powder on diabetic symptoms, anthropometric parameters and blood pressure of non insulin dependent male diabetics. *Ethno–Med.* 2009, 3(1): 5–9.

Koul O, Wahab S, editors. *Neem: Today and in the New Millenium.* Kluwer Academic Publishers. 2004.

Kumar S, Suresh PK, Vijayababu MR, Arunkumar A, Arunakaran J. Anticancer effects of ethanolic neem leaf extract on prostate cancer cell line (PC–3). *J Ethnopharmacol.* 2006, 105(1–2):246–50.

Liu Y, Chen G, Chena Y, Linb J. Inclusion complexes of azadirachtin with native and methylated cyclodextrins: solubilization and binding ability. *Bioorganic & Medicinal Chemistry.* 2005, 13:4037–4042.

Mandal–Ghosh I, Chattopadhyay U, Baral R. Neem leaf preparation enhances Th1 type immune response and anti–tumor immunity against breast tumor associated antigen. *Cancer Immun.* 2007, 7:8.

Mbah AU, Udeinya IJ, Shu EN, Chijioke CP, Nubila T, Udeinya F, Muobuike A, Mmuobieri A, Obioma MS. Fractionated neem leaf extract is safe and increases CD4+ cell levels in HIV/AIDS patients. *Am J Ther.* 2007, 14(4):369–74.

Miaoulis, Nick. Neem farmer and founder of Abaco Neem. Personal interviews. 2009–2012.

Mordue (Luntz) JA, Nisbet A. Azadirachtin from the neem tree Azadirachta indica: its action against insects. *An. Soc. Entomol. Brasil.* 2000, 29(4): 615–632.

Morovati M, Mahmoudi M, Ghazi–Khansari M, Khalil Aria A, Jabbari L. Sterility and abortive effects of the commercial neem (Azadirachta indica A. Juss.) extract NeemAzal– T/S® on female rat (Rattus norvegicus). *Turk J Zool.* 2008, 32:155–162.

Neem: A Tree for Solving Global Problems. Report of an Ad hoc Panel of the Board on Science and Technology for International Development. National Research Council. National Academy Press. 1992.

Neem Foundation website. Accessed March 16, 2009. http://www.Neemfoundation.org.

Norton, Ellen and Jean Putz. *Neem: India's Miraculous Healing Plant.* Healing Arts Press. 2000.

Pai MR, Acharya LD, Udupa N. Evaluation of antiplaque activity of Azadirachta indica leaf extract gel–a 6–week clinical study. *J Ethnopharmacol.* 2004, 90(1):99–103.

Paterson, Pamela. *Neem: Medicinal and Environmental Benefits.* 2012.

Peshin R, Dhawan AK, editors. *Integrated Pest Management: Innovation–Development Process.* Springer Science+Business Media B.V. 2009.

Prashant GM, Chandu GN, Murulikrishna KS, Shafiulla MD. The effect of mango and neem extract on four organisms causing dental caries: Streptococcus mutans, Streptococcus salivavius, Streptococcus mitis, and Streptococcus sanguis: an in vitro study. *Indian J Dent Res.* 2007, 18(4):148–51.

Roy MK, Kobori M, Takenaka M, Nakahara K, Shinmoto H, Isobe S, Tsushida T. Antiproliferative effect on human cancer cell lines after treatment with nimbolide extracted from an edible part of the neem tree (Azadirachta indica). *Phytother Res.* 2007, 21(3):245–50.

Roy MK, Kobori M, Takenaka M, Nakahara K, Shinmoto H, Tsushida T. Inhibition of colon cancer (HT–29) cell proliferation by a triterpenoid isolated from Azadirachta indica is accompanied by cell cycle arrest and up–regulation of p21. *Planta Med.* 2006, 72(10):917–23.

Sharma SK, SaiRam M, Ilavazhagan G, Devendra K, Shivaji SS, Selvamurthy W. Mechanism of action of NIM–76: a novel vaginal contraceptive from neem oil. *Contraception.* 1996, 54(6):373–8.

Sperber Haas, Sheila, editor. *Neem: A hands–on guide to one of the world's most versatile herbs.*

Bibliography

Subapriya R, Nagini S. Medicinal properties of neem leaves: a review. *Curr Med Chem Anticancer Agents.* 2005, 5(2):149–6.

Talwar GP, Raghuvanshi P, Misra R, Mukherjee S, Shah S. Plant immunomodulators for termination of unwanted pregnancy and for contraception and reproductive health. *Immunol Cell Biol.* 1997, 75(2):190–2.

University of Delaware website. Pesticide Safety. Accessed August 9, 2009.

Vanka A, Tandon S, Rao SR, Udupa N, Ramkumar P. The effect of indigenous neem Azadirachta indica mouth wash on Streptococcus mutans and lactobacilli growth. *Indian J Dent Res.* 2001, 12(3):133–44.

Vatandoost H, Hanafi–Bojd AA. Laboratory evaluation of 3 repellents against Anopheles stephensi in the Islamic Republic of Iran. *East Mediterr Health J.* 2008, 14(2):260–7.

Veitch, GE, Beckmann E, Burke BJ, Boyer A, Maslen SL, Ley SV. Synthesis of azadirachtin: a long but successful journey. Angew. *Chem. Int. Ed.* 2007, 46:7629–7632.

Weil, Andrew, M.D. Natural Health, Natural Medicine. *The Complete Guide to Wellness and Self–Care for Optimum Health.* Houghton Mifflin Company. 2004.

Wolinsky LE, Mania S, Nachnani S, Ling S. The inhibiting effect of aqueous Azadirachta indica (Neem) extract upon bacterial properties influencing in vitro plaque formation. *J Dent Res.* 1996, 75(2):816–22.

About the Author

Pamela Paterson, a neem tea drinker, also uses neem for her skin, teeth, and immune system. When she is not consuming neem, she is an author, consultant, college instructor, and speaker.

Pamela has written hundreds of articles, papers, and books in over 30 subject areas. The topics she writes about ranges from business to science to health, and everything in between.

She has a bachelor's degree in journalism and a master's degree in science from the University of Maryland. Pamela was recently inducted into the same honor society as Jimmy Carter, Hilary Rodham Clinton, and Linus C. Pauling.

Pamela lives in Toronto, Canada, and works globally helping people with their writing projects. More information is available at www.writertypes.com.

Index

A
Abaco Neem
    fauna 10
    flora 10
    founder 9
    information center 37
    product chart 39
    starting 9
    story 9
    tour 37
agricultural benefits 33
AIDS 29
Albury, Albert 9
antioxidant 27
aspirin, toxicity 15
azadirachtin
    chemical synthesis 27
    main chemical 13

B
benefits
    agricultural 33
    environment 33
    neem 47

C
cancer 28
chemistry
    azadirachtin 13
    neem 13
    neem oil 13
chicken farm 33
compounds, active 13
contraception 29

D
dental care 28
diabetes 29
Dr. Oz 4

E
environmental benefits 33
Environmental Protection Agency 15
EPA 15
erosion control 33

F
Fleisher, Mitchell 15, 17

H
health benefits, pets 31
health problems
    discussed 27
    neem-treated 17, 47
HIV 29

M
mahogany, cousin of 11

N
National Research Council 4
neem 17
    about 11
    age 12
    altitude 11
    benefits 47
    chemistry 13
    climate 11
    fruit 13
    fruit quantities 12
    fruit, picture 13
    habitat 11
    indoor growing 54
    locations 11
    pollination 12
    remedies 17
    scientific proof 27
    toxicity 15
    tree planting 53

Index

neem flowers
    picture 12
Neem Foundation 15
neem oil, chemistry 13
neem-treated conditions 47
Norton, Ellen 4

O
oral care 28
Oz, Mehmet 4

P
parasite control 33
pest control 34
pesticides 34
    future 35
    home 35
    outlook 35
pet health 31
pet health, remedies 32
pharmacological compounds 13
planting
    indoors 54
    tree 53
pregnancy 29
products, Abaco Neem 39

R
remedies
    list of 17
    pets 32
    product chart 39

S
salt, toxicity 15
science of neem 27
skin disorders 29
soil enhancer 33

T
toxicity
    aspirin 15
    neem 15
    table salt 15

U
ulcers 30

W
Weil, Andrew 4
World Organization of Natural Medicine 10

Made in the USA
Charleston, SC
27 January 2013